To my parents for their love and support.

TABLE OF CONTENTS

INTRODUCTION

I have been researching Chronic Lyme Disease (CLD) and Multiple Systemic Infectious Disease Syndrome (MSIDS) for five years and would like to share what I've learned with you now. If you have been suffering from CLD or MSIDS and are looking to understand how your metabolism can make or break your treatment, then this book is for you. But first, why should you listen to me?

I don't want to fight with you. I am just an observer who is up to date on who is warring with whom, while I watch and eat my popcorn. I find correlational research and case studies conducted by university hospitals, clinics, and labs to be far more relevant than articles on Mercola.com and the like. Even more interesting to me, however, is the growing body of experimental research that is available online because of people who are voluntarily turning themselves into guinea pigs and sharing their results on forums. I sure have. When you have a disease that doctors don't fully understand, experimentation is inevitable.

There are a lot of Lyme *professionnels* (the fancy French way of saying professionals), from Buhner, to Cowden, to Klinghardt, to Horowitz, and I've studied up on all of them. I have my own super team of infectious disease doctors to learn from as well. I'd like to say that two heads are better than one, but add all these opinions together and what you get is a chaotic pile of controversial shitake. Everyone seems to have a different protocol, a different diet and/or a different strategy for getting better. Some of these strategies include quick fixes such as antibiotics. Some of them however, like fasting, are so intense they require retirement and full-time rest.

I've personally tried some of these popular drugs, herbs, diets, and suggestions from the *professionnels* and you know what I've realized? Lyme disease is friggin' complex. There is no miracle cure.

Furthermore, the word "Lyme" has come to represent more than Borrelia burgdorferi. Lyme disease is controversial. Some doctors do not even recognize it. Personally, I am not concerned with the politics or semantics. I am not affiliated with any of the sources referenced here and this book is not here to prove that you have Lyme. Rather, *it is a book for anyone who has an infection, in general, and cannot seem to get rid of it because his or her immune system and supportive therapies are not keeping up*. This book was formulated in the strong belief that there are more than two kinds of infections - acute infections that kill you and acute infections that go away. In this book, I will use the word "Lyme" to represent not only Borrelia, but also chronic infections in general.

My Story

My doctor tested me five years ago for the Canadian ELISA, which came back negative. I continued seeing specialists such as neurologists, endocrinologists, gastroenterologists, ENT doctors, and cardiologists. I had all sorts of testing done, among them ultrasounds, CT scans, endoscopies, biopsies, and the list goes on. Don't get me started on how much blood work I've had done: enough to make a whole new human, I bet. Eventually I stumbled upon a physiatrist, a doc who specializes in musculoskeletal pain. He did blood work for CD57, vitamin D and the Western Blot. And voila! I had a diagnosis! I promptly cried for a day about the thought of ending up in a wheelchair, but then I began my journey to recovery.

Long story short, I had an undiagnosed infection ravaging my body for years before I started treatment. I am very aware of how damaging CLD is to the entire body and how hopeless it can feel to have everything fall apart.

If you found out you had Lyme one week after contracting it, then hurrah! Get your antibiotics and move on. However, CLD has become a tragic reality for many of us who didn't catch it in time; unfortunately, our numbers are growing every year.

I am here to tell you that recovery is not easy; it goes way, *way* beyond antibiotics and low-carb diets. In my personal journey, repairing my body and reducing my infection has required the utmost diligence, patience, optimism and time. But *staying in remission* was what required the most research.

At my worst, I couldn't sort out my words, my short-term memory was shot, and I essentially felt stupid. I couldn't exercise, nay, even walking up the stairs left me dizzy and breathless. I was itchy all over, I felt

electric shocks and sharp pains up and down my limbs
and all over my head. My face was flushed, my body
temperature and blood pressure were dangerously low,
my bowels shut down, my glands hurt, my throat was
chronically sore, *and* I hacked up phlegm like a butt-
smoking truck driver. Some of my friends stuck with me
through it all, but others, not so much. I felt like a leper
and I desperately missed carbs, which I had cut out of my
diet almost completely.

In the course of a single year, I tried a juice fast,
followed by a very low-carb diet concoction, an
autoimmune paleo diet, a low FODMAPS diet, the GAPS
diet, and a diet low in polyunsaturated fats. All the while
I was on antimicrobials, enzymes and chelators and
having intravenous therapies like the Myer's Cocktail and
glutathione pushes. While my symptoms did improve, I
could not get off the antimicrobials without my
symptoms returning.

I've spent 5 years creeping health forums and
researching multiple aspects of anatomy and infectious
diseases. This research has led me to experiment with my
own health, trying drastic and even life threatening
treatments such as IV chelation. It has also led me to
rethink many times the usefulness as well as the problems
caused by various treatments.

**The Game Changer (and Not for the Reason
You'd Think)**

Thanks to a bit of research and a bit of self-
experimentation I stumbled upon something that changed
my way of thinking. It was simple: Manuka honey. I
justified taking a tablespoon of Manuka honey a day for

its high methygloxyl content, which is a hydrogen peroxide producing anti-microbial. I started to feel more energetic, so I added another tablespoon throughout the day. Then another, and another. Eventually, I reached the point where I was ingesting five tablespoons of Manuka honey each day.

At this point, how could I not re-evaluate my low-carb lifestyle? I started adding in a few carbs such as potatoes, fruits, and even refined table sugar *(gasp)*. My energy was better than it had been in years and I actually started up some moderately intense weight-training with no ill effects. My body temperature warmed up, my brain felt sharper, and I could stomach a broader spectrum of foods. More importantly, my immune system became resilient enough to get off the antimicrobials and stay off them.

Why I Am Writing This

If you focus all your energy on killing the bugs I truly don't believe you are seeing the whole picture. I don't want to convince you to throw your antibiotics down the drain (although I did), but if your body is not responding to the antibiotics, or if you are responding well and want to further optimize your health, then I have a lot to share with you, my ill friend.

I am only a single case study, but this book is not about my protocol. It's rather a summary of the information I've collected from physiology, anatomy and drug metabolism textbooks, as well as articles and books on chronic infections and immunity. These resources have helped me realize that it's not just tick-slaying that can help reduce infections. I saw real improvements from investigating the following aspects of health:

1. Metabolism

2. Immunity and the lymphatic system

3. Gut health

4. Hematology

5. Biofilm and persisters

6. Liver health and detoxification

7. Sleep, stress and hormones

8. Genetics

9. Antigens

10. Perspective

I am writing *this* book with a focus on the metabolism. I think that metabolism is significant enough to the recovery process to merit its own book. Once you have finished this book, I believe you will agree.

I know you didn't ask for a chronic illness. Fun fact: me, neither. But recovery is a *good* thing and good things don't come easy. Let's feel well again and stay that way.

Solution

The point of this book is to give you an introductory understanding of metabolism, something I believe is underrated in the Lyme recovery process. This book can be useful as a science-based, affordable, practical, and – dare I say – fun way to get into remission and stay there.

Your metabolism takes time to repair but it is oh-so-necessary for remission and good health. My immune system is a lot stronger now that my thyroid, body temperature, and cellular energy production are functioning within a therapeutic range. It is certainly much stronger than when I was suffering and sugar- and carb-free. What a revelation to realize that "feeding the bugs" feeds me, too!

What Is Different About This Book?

I won't go into a million case-studies, but I will correlate and compare different professional theories about medical modalities. I will also make some medical jargon more comprehensible to help you better understand your metabolism.

This Book Will Address:

- Introductory anatomy that everyone should know

- Why metabolism is important and how it slows due to infections

- How poor metabolic function undermines treatment

- Why Lyme patients are generally underfed

- Food, supplements and practices that speed and slow metabolism and your infection fighting power

- How adverse drug reactions are related to metabolism

- The importance of mitochondria in energy production

- How solely focusing on "bug killing" can worsen your condition

I was at rock bottom. The combination of an out-of-control infection and the wrong treatments put me in a bad place, both physically and mentally. Like I said, patience, diligence, optimism and research got me to where I am now. What I learned was that killing the bugs was not enough and it could even *cause* harm without at the same time providing support to my gut, hormones, liver, metabolism, and everything else "me."

This book is going to zero in on metabolism, a system that ought to be in a healthy condition if we want to *stay* in remission. By fixing your metabolism, you can modulate your immune responses and increase valuable energy needed to fight chronic infections.

CHAPTER 1: METABOLISM FOR DUMMIES

What Is Metabolism?

Nutrients in your food are digested and absorbed by your cells. That's metabolism in a nutshell. However, there are a few more facets to metabolism I would like to review with you. I've tried to summarize it in a way that removes the technical stuff (like how many molecules glucose splits into when catabolized), but I still think it is important to know how on earth food works to energize us. There is a lot of information to absorb in this chapter but please don't skip it, as the terminology reviewed here will come up a lot throughout the book.

What Happens After Foods Break Down?

After nutrients are absorbed they are used to burn energy, as calories. This is called *catabolism*. In catabolism, cells break down fat, protein and carbs to release energy. This energy can be stored, given off as heat or used to maintain body temperature. Catabolism generates *ATP*, the molecule that helps release energy from your cells.

If catabolism breaks things down, *anabolism* builds things up. Catabolism is like jumping on a pile of grapes, whereas anabolism is like making grapes into wine. Catabolic energy fuels anabolism.

In anabolism, energy is stored or used to build and repair the body. Chemical reactions within the cells synthesize new materials for cellular use by making large molecules out of smaller ones. So, while in catabolism carbs are broken down into cute lil' glucose molecules, in anabolism, glucose molecules link together to make larger glycogen molecules.

We should all give a big thanks to our *mitochondria* for making these processes happen. Our mitochondria, which are found in most cells, are kind of like furnaces – they burn glucose to create ATP. The better your mitochondria work, the more energy they can pull out of food and the air. Stay tuned. In Chapter 10 you will discover how to increase your mitochondrial content.

Fuel for Life

Energy from food is measured in what we know as calories. A calorie is the amount of energy needed to raise the temperature of one gram of water by one degree, Celsius. A gram of protein contains 4 calories. The same applies to carbs. A gram of fat is more energy dense, at 9 calories per gram. We use calories to move, to support basal metabolism and to produce heat. Because of this, try to think of calories as your fuel source, not your enemy.

Basal metabolism is the minimum (or base) amount of calories necessary to maintain simple body functions. Basal metabolism is highest in men, young people, those with a lot of muscle mass and people with fevers. Hormones such as thyroxine, growth hormone, and epinephrine also increase your basal metabolism. For the average person, more than 60% of your energy is used to maintain your basal metabolism. In Chapter 7 you will find out why sick people need even *more* calories.

We produce heat to process food as well as to maintain a healthy body temperature. Your body temperature affects how well enzymes function, and in chapter 8 you will discover why healthy enzymes are necessary for both liver and drug metabolism.

What Is Being Metabolized?

Carbs, fats and proteins break down into smaller molecules before our cells can use them. After digestion, these molecules make their way into our cells and their mitochondria, where they are used as energy.

Each of these energy sources breaks down differently. Carbs break down into sugars such as glucose. Proteins break down into amino acids and fats break down into fatty acids and glycerol. In addition, these each have different functions.

Carbs

Besides being tasty, carbs catabolize into glucose in the liver. Catabolizing glucose takes ATP, which converts the glucose into *pyruvic acid* and even more ATP than it took to convert it (fun fact: it takes 2 ATP molecules to catabolize glucose, but produces 4, giving you a net gain of 2 ATP molecules). Remember, ATP is the molecule that helps release energy.

Pyruvic acid is the version of glucose that can squeeze inside your mitochondria. Once pyruvic acid enters the mitochondria it produces *acetyl-CoA*. In something called the citric acid cycle, acetyl-CoA produces carbon dioxide, which we breathe out, as well as ATP and heat.

The most important thing to take away here is that *ATP helps carbs break down into glucose, and that glucose goes through a life cycle ending in the production of carbon dioxide and even more ATP than it took to break it down initially.*

Your blood glucose level rises when glucose is absorbed through the digestive tract. But don't get your diabetes-fearing panties in a bundle; your liver removes glucose from the bloodstream, storing it as glycogen. Only if your glycogen storage is full, will excess glucose be converted into fat.

Your blood glucose is lowest after not eating for a long time. When your blood sugar is too low, you have glycogen stored in the liver that your body can use as a glucose substitute. Pretty helpful. The trouble arises when your glycogen stores run out; without glucose or glycogen available, your body must convert protein into glucose to stay alive – and this require a large surge of cortisol. Inflammation is a likely outcome. Personally, I'd rather get my glucose from something yum than be inflamed while converting my proteins into glucose on a miserable carbless diet.

Proteins

"If cows could fly, I'd bet their wings would taste delicious" – bad meat joke.

Proteins catabolize into *amino acids*. They're absorbed by your small intestines. From there they enter your hepatic portal circulation to reach your liver, and finally are sent into general circulation throughout your body to become available to your cells.

Amino acids build new tissues and repair damaged ones. They also synthesize hemoglobin, hormones, enzymes, and plasma proteins. Your body does not store amino acids for later use, so a daily supply supports these processes. They *can* be used as energy if there are insufficient amounts of carbs and fats in the diet, but their primary purpose is for use in the above anabolic processes.

Deamination is the catabolism of amino acids. This process removes an amino group from the amino acid to form a keto acid and ammonia. Ammonia is toxic to cells, so the liver converts it to urea, which is excreted in the urine. Some keto acids convert to pyruvic acid or acetyl-CoA; others convert to glucose and fat molecules if there is an excess of amino acids.

Fats

"Dear Lord, if you can't make me skinny please make my friends fat" – bad fat joke.

Your brain cannot run on fat, but the rest of your body can. Fats also provide essential fatty acids, absorb fat soluble vitamins (A, K, D, and E), serve as building blocks for cell membranes and myelin, and provide insulation. If you overeat fats they can store as *adipose tissue*, a concentrated energy source.

Fats convert into *glycerol* and *fatty acids*. Glycerol enters the citric acid cycle to produce ATP, carbon dioxide and water. Fatty acids convert into acetyl-CoA. If there is an excess of acetyl-CoA then ketone bodies form. Ketones are usually acidic, so the body can become too acidic when you have an excess of acetyl-CoA.

Chapter Takeaways:

- Carbs are tasty.

- Carbs, fats and proteins breakdown into smaller molecules before our cells can use them.

- Carbs catabolize into glucose, which gives our mitochondria energy.

- Proteins catabolize into amino acids, which are used for anabolic processes like synthesizing hemoglobin, hormones, enzymes and plasma proteins.

- Fats catabolize into glycerol and fatty acids, both of which go through the same citric acid cycle that carbs do, but at a slower rate.

- Excess fat can become concentrated fat storage called adipose tissue.

That's the long-story-short of metabolism. I hope you learned something. Now let's talk about why this applies to you.

CHAPTER 2: LYME AFFECTS METABOLISM

If you suffer from fatigue, brain fog, constipation, food sensitivities, frequent urination, insomnia, cold hands and feet or a temperature under 97.8 degrees Fahrenheit, not to mention Lyme, you probably have a slow metabolism.

Metabolism is what helps your body turn food, water, air, vitamins, and minerals into energy for your cells. Your *metabolic rate* is how fast your cells use energy. A low metabolic rate reduces your immunity, slows digestion, releases stress hormones, and worsens leaky gut, ultimately reducing immunity and increasing inflammation. A fast metabolism manifests in many ways, such as a moderate to high pulse rate, an abundance of fidgety energy, or a high body temperature. Think toddlers on sugar.

Lyme Slows Metabolism

Chronic infections are chronic stressors. Stress raises the stress hormone cortisol. Chronically elevated cortisol affects leptin, which is important to your thyroid function. Do you have a low body temperature? Is sleep unsatisfying? Ya' tired? No sex drive? Pee a lot? You may have the metabolism of an 80 year old, as I did. A weak metabolism kind of goes hand in hand with chronic infections.

Slow Metabolism Slows Recovery

In Matt Stone's words, metabolism works like this:

"When metabolism falls, your sex hormone production falls (infertility, loss of sex drive, loss of period, erectile dysfunction, PMS). When metabolism falls, your youth hormone (growth hormone) falls, and you lose your ability to build muscle tissue, perform athletically, and you lose muscle tissue. When metabolism falls, your rate of fat burning decreases and your body starts to manufacture more fat out of the food you eat. This causes a rise in triglycerides in your blood leading to insulin resistance (the precursor to metabolic syndrome and type 2 diabetes), increased appetite, increased storage of the food you eat into fat cells, and so forth. When metabolism falls you produce more estrogen (both men and women) and the opposing hormones testosterone and progesterone are produced in smaller quantities."

In short, a lousy metabolism throws the body off balance to a point where we physically may not have as much "fight" left in us.

Furthermore, when metabolism falls, the body becomes an environment prone to inflammation.

The immune system releases proteins called cytokines. Some are anti-inflammatory (Yay!) and some are pro-inflammatory (Boo!). Acute inflammation is created as a healing response. However, Lyme and its co-infections *chronically* produce   pro-inflammatory cytokines (Double-boo!) and suppress anti-inflammatory cytokines.

Chronic inflammation is what breaks down tissue such as collagen so the bacteria can use it as food (mmm…food). Let me repeat that: **Thanks to *chronic* inflammation, bacteria can *eat* our catabolized body tissue.** This is where muscle wasting and heart and brain problems come in.

So a weak metabolism makes it hard to fight infections. And the inflammation produced makes it easy for infections to find food sources. To come full circle, chronic infections allow metabolism to fall further. This is a bad cycle to enter.

Here are some examples of the role inflammation plays in infections:

- Mycoplasma depends on inflammation and immune dysregulation to thrive.

- Babesia and Bartonella depend on inflammation and immune dysregulation to infect red blood cells.

- Ehrlichia and Anaplasma depend on inflammation and immune dysregulation to infect white blood cells.

- Lyme depends on inflammation to deteriorate collagen into bug meal.

How to Not Be Bug Meal

Strengthen your immune system, inhibit inflammation and protect red blood cells, and the bugs begin to die without even obsessing over killing them.

Take away inflammation by doing things like improving your metabolism and you make your body not only less arthritic and feeble, but you clean out the infection's all-you-can-eat buffet of inflammation. Killing the bugs with antimicrobials may be a part of the healing process, but nothing will help your body *keep the infection at bay* like a strong immune system. Antibiotics do a lot, but they sure as hell don't strengthen your immunity.

Chapter Takeaways:

It doesn't make sense to fixate on killing the bugs when your metabolism can barely tolerate the food and herbs needed to eliminate them and to repair your body. *However*, if you can strengthen your metabolism then good things like this happen:

- Your digestive engines work faster and you have fewer problems with constipation and food sensitivities. The hormone gastrin increases, so processing hard-to-digest foods becomes a lot easier.

- Better digested food = more nutrients for your cells to metabolize. Nourished cells give you a better quality of life in countless ways.

- Your thyroid functions better and your thyroid has a lot of say in the health of your liver.

- Cortisol and insulin resistance decrease and improved glucose clearance follows.

- Your body temperature goes up, which warms you and increases enzymatic processes. The better your enzymes function, the more your foods, drugs, and toxins are metabolized and detoxified.

- Mitochondria work better, making you feel physically stronger.

- Your constitution gets stronger and you start working *with* your body instead of *against* it.

CHAPTER 3: ADRENAL FATIGUE: THE BEGINNING OF THE END

Adrenal Fatigue Syndrome is caused by stress, imbalances of the Hypothalamic-Pituitary-Adrenal (HPA) Axis, nervous system problems, metabolic problems, and poor immunity. Adrenal fatigue produces countless issues including fatigue, allergies, frequent infections, anxiety, poor concentration, and insomnia.

Adrenals at a Glance

The adrenal glands release epinephrine and norepinephrine, hormones responsible for the fight-or-flight response. The adrenal cortex produces mineralocorticoids (like aldosterone), androgens (like pregnenalone) and glucocorticoids (like cortisol).

Let's Define These Terms:

Aldosterone regulates the balance of sodium and potassium in our cells and in consequence affects our blood pressure.

Pregnenalone generates cortisol and the sex hormones DHEA, testosterone, estrogen, and progesterone. As my home-girls know, you can go totally cray-cray when these are out of whack.

Finally, *cortisol* fights stress, regulates blood sugar and is secreted as an anti-inflammatory response.

As your stress level increases, more cortisol is produced. The HPA axis creates Adrenal Corticotropic Hormone (ACTH) in order to adjust your cortisol levels, which in turn allows cholesterol to be turned into pregnenalone, the precursor to many hormones.

Normally, your cortisol is highest at 8am, and drops twice, from 9:30am to 11:30am and again from 3:30pm to 5:30pm. Your cortisol levels are lowest from 12:30am to 4:30am.

So When You Are About to Outrun a Tiger:

1. Your sympathetic nervous system is activated, which means

2. ACTH is released from your pituitary gland, triggering the release of epinephrine and cortisol.

3. Your blood pressure increases, your muscles tense, and glucose increases in your blood to help you fight (or "flight", if you're a lil' bitch).

4. Digestion slows because your blood has moved to support your muscles and your heart.

5. You pee yourself so you can get rid of any extra weight. Ha!

You Can't Run Forever

If internal, external, or mental perceptions of stress are chronic, your adrenal glands can't keep up with your body's need for cortisol. Adrenal fatigue is the result.

Here are some consequences of chronic stress:

- Your body converts pregnenalone into cortisol while neglecting the production of sex hormones. Estrogen dominance occurs, messing up your menstrual cycle and causing infertility.

- Once your hormones are imbalanced, secretory IgA (your cellular defence), NK cells and T-lymphocytes are reduced, so bacterial and viral infections become harder to fight off and easier to catch.

- The low blood pressure that follows can leave you feeling like a zombie and may give you vertigo when you change positions.

- Hypothyroidism and poor metabolism also follow.

- Postural orthostatic tachycardia syndrome, more commonly known as POTS, is a symptom of Lyme but it's also a symptom of weak adrenals. Sweating profusely or not at all, thermal imbalances, and postural hypotension (a form of low blood pressure that makes you dizzy when you stand up) can occur. POTS was personally my most crippling symptom.

- The Ovarian-Adrenal-Thyroid (OAT) Axis can become imbalanced. The ovaries, adrenals and thyroid depend on one another. When one is affected by stress, all three can become affected. For example, progesterone production, normally the work of the adrenal glands, comes to a halt in favor of cortisol production. This leads to estrogen dominance, which raises thyroid-binding proteins and lowers T3 and T4. Like me, it's a delicate ecosystem.

Treating Adrenal Fatigue

When you have a chronic infection, your body is stressed enough as is. Do what you can to remove stressors wherever possible. Here are a few things that may help:

- Go to sleep by 10pm. This is the time your adrenals work hardest to repair your body.

- If you wake up easily throughout the night, consider a sleep aid concoction. Mine is simple: magnesium and B6 with a snack if I'm hungry.

- Limit stimulants. If you drink coffee, drink it when your cortisol is low - 9:30am to 11:30am or 3:30pm to 5:30pm.

- Breathe and stretch. Gradually work your way up to yoga or lifting weights. Among other benefits, exercise boosts happy hormones and confidence, thereby reducing stress. Overdoing exercise, however, can worsen adrenal fatigue. More on this in Chapter 10.

- Supplement with Vitamin C, B vitamins, Vitamin D, and Magnesium to support your adrenals. Food and sunlight are superior to pills, if you can get them.

- Support your digestion, as digesting food takes energy. Get adequate energy by increasing caloric intake and sleep. Betaine HCl is a digestive aid that may increase stomach acidity, if hypochlorhydria is an issue for you, but the scientific evidence to support this claim is lacking. That said, many people believe it helps them. Conversely, if you produce too much stomach acid, limiting fatty foods may benefit you. This topic merits a whole other book, but let me just add that digestive support will vary from individual to individual.

- Adaptogens are controversial. Research the pros and cons of them before use. The more severe your adrenal fatigue, the more likely these herbs will act as stimulants and make you crash. More on this in Chapter 4.

- Consider adrenal cortex supplements for mild adrenal fatigue.

- Research hydrocortisone for severely low adrenal fatigue. Caution: Hydrocortisone suppresses the HPA feedback loop, and can lower your sex hormones and calcium levels.

- Eat breakfast to fuel your body. Today may not be the best time to try intermittent fasting or ketogenic diets. A lot of people with weak adrenals are borderline hypoglycemic. Eat protein and fat, which fuel the body slowly and sufficiently until your next meal. Eat carbs at the end of your meals to avoid sugar spikes.

- If you have high blood pressure and ACTH, reduce your salt intake. If you have low blood pressure and ACTH, increase your salt intake.

- Stay calm, be patient and listen to your body.

CHAPTER 4: A SLOW METABOLISM MESSES WITH YOUR THYROID

Hypothyroidism is just the worst if you have Lyme.

Without addressing the thyroid, detoxification is undermined, estrogen dominance and anemia can occur, and inflammation and infections can take over our bodies. If you are hypothyroid, other things can be affected like the hypothalamus, the pituitary gland, the thymus gland, as well as your liver, heart, nerves, muscles and enzymes. Let's get into the details.

But First, How Does the Thyroid Work? Well:

1. The hypothalamus sends Thyroid Releasing Hormone (TRH) to the pituitary gland.

2. The pituitary gland releases TSH to the thymus gland.

3. TSH stimulates TPO activity to use iodine and hydrogen peroxide to create (mostly) T4 and (very little) T3. T4 is unusable so it has to be converted into more T3 elsewhere (ahem, the liver).

4. The thyroid hormones hop onto thyroid-binding proteins to catch a ride through the blood stream before jumping off to find cells - hence they become "free" hormones.

5. The liver converts T4 into T3. The thyroid only produces 7% of T3 you need, so your liver converts more via conjugation pathways. The heart, muscles and nerves convert T4 into T3 in lesser quantities. Cells in these organs convert T4 to T3 by using an enzyme, tetraidothyronine 5' deiodinase, which removes one molecule of iodine from T4 (T4 minus 1 = T3…woah).

6. 20% of your T3 becomes active in the intestines, if the gut is healthy. (Antibiotics can hurt the gut. Thus, antibiotics dampen thyroid function, too…just another reason they suck).

7. T3 enters the nucleus of each cell where it turns genes on or off, influencing their destiny to do things such as generate heat.

Now, here are ten reasons why hypothyroidism is the worst thing for Lyme disease.

Reason 1: Gastrointestinal Function

Hypothyroidism slows the time it takes for food to move through the GI tract, increasing infections, inflammation, nutrient deficiency and food intolerances.

Back in Chapter 2 we talked about how inflammation and nutrient deficiency can stunt your recovery.

Reason 2: Liver Function

Hypothyroidism makes the liver sluggish. We *need* a healthy liver for metabolizing T4, our sex hormones and all sorts of other hormones. We need it for filtering toxins like infectious disease by-products and antibiotics, and for cleaning the blood. Once the liver becomes sluggish, it makes hypothyroidism worse, which only makes the liver more sluggish, which makes hypothyroidism worse, which…you get the picture. It's an endless cycle. Without a healthy liver, your efforts at detoxifying can be pointless until the thyroid is addressed.

Hypothyroidism also elevates homocysteine by compromising the liver's ability to manage this amino acid. Too much homocysteine may increase heart disease, dementia and Neurogenerative diseases.

Reason 3: Growth Hormone Production

It takes a healthy amount of thyroid hormones to make Growth Hormone (GH). GH helps regenerate cells, so good luck building up muscle when it's low. Deconditioned muscles have less mitochondria to work with than strong healthy ones, as we will discuss more in Chapter 10.

Reason 4: Fat Burning Abilities

Hypothyroidism slows your metabolism. It shuts down sites on your cells that respond to lipase, an enzyme that metabolizes fat. We ought to be able to burn fat for energy. But if we cannot, then we can only rely on sugar for energy. With hypothyroidism, fat does not get burned effectively, no matter how much you exercise. It only accumulates, making you – for lack of a better word – fat.

Reason 5: Insulin and Glucose Metabolism

Your brain uses most of your body's glucose, so when your glucose metabolism sucks, your brain function sucks, too.

With hypothyroidism two things happen: glucose is absorbed more slowly and glucose is harder to eliminate. Not enough sugar becomes available for energy. To compensate for the resulting low energy state, the adrenals pump out stress hormones to activate the release of – oh, crap! – even *more* glucose into the blood stream.

This glucose is no easier to eliminate or absorb than the other glucose you have floating around. You can end up with a busload of glucose in your blood that is not being used properly. Your stress hormones keep activating the release of glucose from your liver in confusion, and your adrenals become exhausted. The problem isn't too little glucose in your blood; it's too little glucose getting into your cells.

I also have to wonder if the overload of stagnant blood glucose is feeding the infection, despite all your efforts to eat sugar-free…

Reason 6: Cholesterol

With hypothyroidism, you can produce fat quicker than you can burn it, driving up cholesterol. Paired with a weak liver that can't metabolize the fat, more LDL accumulates in the blood.

Reason 7: Estrogen Production

Estrogen must be made water soluble in the liver, but with hypothyroidism, the liver may be too weak to eliminate excess estrogen. Too much estrogen contributes to ovarian, breast and prostate cancer. It also creates too many thyroid-binding proteins, so the T4 and T3 never get out of their thyroid-binding taxi-cabs.

Reason 8: Progesterone Production

The thyroid and progesterone are a team. Progesterone improves the signalling of thyroid receptors and stimulates TPO production. This is why temperature normalizes when women are ovulating. However, when estrogen stagnates in the body because the liver is not filtering estrogen out fast enough, estrogen dominance occurs. This reduces the progesterone-to-estrogen ratio in the body. A sluggish pituitary gland, birth control pills, menopause, or adrenal fatigue due to infection can also create estrogen dominance.

A healthy thyroid can sensitize your cells to progesterone so that they can readily pick it up. But when the progesterone receptors on your cells are not exposed frequently enough to thyroid hormones, your progesterone is locked out of your cells, even though there may be tons of it in your bloodstream.

If you don't have enough progesterone, it throws off your thyroid function. If you don't have enough thyroid hormones, this in turn will throw off your progesterone balance and the vicious cycle (not to mention estrogen dominance) begins.

Reason 9: Low Stomach Acid

The hormone gastrin increases stomach acidity and stimulates the gallbladder and pancreas to aid digestion. Gastrin production somewhat depends on thyroid health. With hypothyroidism you can expect low stomach acidity, which may result in hindered absorption of nutrients, inflammation and infection.

Reason 10: Anemia

Lastly, hypothyroidism creates anemia from deficiencies in B12, folic acid and iron. When stomach acidity is low, so is absorption of valuable nutrients.

As you can see, there are a lot of good reasons to take care of your thyroid if you want to stay in remission.

Foods That Suppress Thyroid Function

There are many antimicrobial herbs, supplements, and foods that suppress thyroid function. Let's look at some things you may be doing that can add insult to thyroid-injury.

Dietary Considerations:

- Gluten intolerance is common in Hashimoto's patients. Gliadin, a component of gluten, has a molecular structure similar to your thyroid hormones. If gliadin gets into the blood stream, your immune system tracks it to get rid of the intruder. But since gliadin resembles your thyroid molecules, the immune system may attack these, as well.

- Get adequate protein, selenium, and tyrosine in your diet.

- There is tyrosine in eggs, saltwater fish, turkey, chicken, cottage cheese, hard cheese, pork, gamey meat, beef, and sea vegetables.

- Polyunsaturated fats may suppress thyroid function. Boost thyroid and metabolism with saturated oils like coconut oil and ghee.

- Be aware that goitrogens, some herbs, and toxins such as bromine, chlorine and fluoride prevent the iodine absorption needed for proper thyroid function.

- Iodine *absorption* is more important than iodine supplementation. Actually, supplementing with iodine can be dangerous. Limit goitrogenic foods; these can block your thyroid's ability to absorb iodine. Goitrogens are found in broccoli, cabbage, kale, spinach, sweet potatoes, canola, millet, tapioca, mustard, strawberries and more. You can cook these in water and dump the water to reduce goitrogens.

Herbs That Suppress Thyroid Function:

- The antimicrobials Japanese knotweed, isatis, and sida acuta

- The sleep herbs valerian root, passion flower, and motherwort

- Green tea due to ECGC and fluoride content

- Quercetin in large doses

- Cannabis, possibly

- Curcumin, possibly

- Others, probably. Look into how your medications might influence thyroid health.

Some Herbs to Consider:

- Nettle assists with T4-T3 conversion.

- Bacopa increases T4 though it may not improve conversion to T3.

- Guggul improves T4-T3 conversion, cholesterol and metabolic rate, though it may be estrogenic.

- Like antibiotics, I think adaptogens should be pulsed, if used at all. Rhodiola is good for the thyroid and HPA axis. I take this every day for half the month along with vitex, which boosts progesterone. The other half of the month I take maca, another adaptogen.

- Since 80% of thyroid hormone conversion takes place in the liver, herbs that support the liver, such as milk thistle, can be used. Not getting hammered off of vodka is a good one, too.

For more info on the above herbs I recommend looking into Stephen Buhner's *Herbal Antibiotics*, or Joey Lott's *Healing Chronic Lyme Disease Naturally*.

It's okay to incorporate these foods and herbs into your life, but be prudent, do your research, and when in doubt, support your thyroid.

CHAPTER 5: NO PERFECT DIET FOR LYME AND METABOLISM

I have been chasing the perfect diet for years. I've had to take into account that I have a couple pathogens to fight off, food sensitivities, endocrine issues like hypothyroidism and estrogen dominance, hematological problems like anemia, and so on. But sick or not, there seems to be evidence to back *every* opposing claim regarding dietary *perfection.*

What I have found in my research is not a perfect diet, but a whole lot of angry people defending their extreme claims and trying to pull beginner-health-seekers into their opposing fads. These diet fads are problematically backed by case studies and empirical evidence, so it is easy to get swept up in low-carb, low-fat, juicing, or the many other "curative" diet trends.

I guess that is how I ended up trying many of these diets to begin with. Once you get sucked in there is a lot of great information that scrolls on endlessly. "Wow", I'd say to myself as I scrolled through the research and testimonials, "*this* diet is established."

Yet when I google various theories, I can find strong evidence to both support *and* oppose every diet I've been on. Keep this in mind if you ever find yourself proselytizing on behalf of a singular expert or diet.

Experimentation, observation and experience may come close to objectifying theories, but they are all influenced by the researcher's beliefs and experiences. Even when there are agreed methods of interpreting data, two scientists using a single set of data can come to very different conclusions.

My Experience

I tried juice fasting for one month first. Juicing gives your stomach time to rest while loading you with phytonutrients and antioxidants. It allows your body to use its energy to repair other bodily systems and gives you time to produce more salivary enzymes that will break down your food once you start eating again. *How sweet is that?*

But fruits and vegetables, though nutrient dense, don't provide us with all the nutrients our bodies need. Strictly juicing deprives you of protein and fat, which are valuable for repair, growth, hormone production, and a whole host of other bodily functions. Also, juicing raw vegetables high in goitrogens may actually undermine your thyroid health.

Then I tried a low-carb paleo diet, of course. If you are sedentary, as many Lyme patients are (though not by choice), then you can live with fewer carbs. What's more, carbs "feed" bacteria in our intestines. *I'd better not eat any carbs if I want to survive this*, I thought at the time. In a resting state our bodies run on fat (lipolysis) anyways. When very low-carb (VLC), our bodies adapt so that we don't need as many carbs, our sugar cravings disappear, we don't get blood sugar spikes, and we start eating rich foods full of saturated fats and cholesterol that are precursors to creating our hormones. I increased my intake of egg yolks which are a great source of choline and selenium, and ghee (or butter) which is your only good source of butyric acid besides starch. In theory, hormone regulation, bug-killing and miraculous health should appear when on this diet. A lot of sick people, not to mention healthy people, are "paleo." Can you say *established*?

But my hormones didn't regulate. My hands and feet were always cold and my progesterone plummeted. Without a working metabolism, my body would never be able to fight off infections without the assistance of drugs. I soon realized that carbs were necessary – nay, carbs were *the answer*. A lot of research suggests that carbs not only fuel our bodies, but they help reduce insulin resistance. Actually, insulin resistance can occur when we deprive ourselves of carbs, because our glycogen stores become depleted in our livers so often that our bodies constantly create glucose to compensate. Our bodies can run on ketones, sure, but our brains NEED glucose. If we exercise (and we *should* exercise, if only for the pro-oxidant and ATP effects we need to boost mitochondrial function), then carbs are essential to help our muscles repair. If we don't have enough for at least that, we will make glucose out of anything – even our own muscles. Along with this muscle wasting, our adrenals become taxed and that hormonal balance we sought after with the VLC diet dies, along with our fatty dreams.

So I kept my protein intake at what it was (.7 grams per pound of body weight), went high-carb, low-fat and got achy hips again. When I added back some fat – no more achy hips.

This is kind of where I'm at now, but I have more unanswered questions than ever. That's a lie, actually. All of my questions have been answered. Every theory I've had has been proven. And that's the problem.

I dare you to google some of these topics and send me an email at yessington@itsnotjustlyme.com with The Objective Truth (good luck):

1. Glucose v.s. fructose v.s. starch as a source of fuel (Mercola thinks fructose is bad; Ray Peat thinks glucose and starch are inferior).

2. Fiber v.s. no fiber (as fiber helps with peristalsis and feeds our microbiome but fiber also feeds bacteria, irritates weak GI tracts and may be estrogenic). Further: soluble fiber v.s. insoluble fiber v.s. both v.s. none.

3. Phytic acid (it's an anti-oxidant) v.s. no phytic acid (it's an anti-nutrient).

4. Sugar for fuel v.s. limiting sugar for killing bacteria.

5. Upon waking: start the day with protein to avoid blood sugar spikes v.s. carbs to "break the fast."

6. Fish oil benefits (omega-3) v.s. fish oil dangers (fish oil oxidizes and goes rancid quickly, and is high in polyunsaturated fats and metals).

7. Polyunsaturated fats (PUFAs) are healthy v.s. PUFA's are unhealthy and oxidize easily.

8. Germ-free guts v.s. healthy microbiomes.

9. Raw v.s. cooked foods.

10. Raw milk v.s. pasteurized milk v.s. eliminating milk.

Then there are the array of **popular diets** to consider:

1. **Traditional Chinese Medicine style diets**, which focus on balance (i.e. "cool" a "hot" body, "wet" a "dry" body, "dry" a "wet" body, and so on).

2. **The Specific Carb Diet**, which advocates simple carbs that are metabolized higher in the GI tract and avoids complex carbs that feed bacteria lower in the digestive tract.

3. **Paleo**, which advocates real foods like meat, animal fats, vegetables, fruits and nuts. Paleo can be broken down into primal (high fat and dairy), low-carb (high fat, no dairy) and in other ways as presented by Chris Kresser, Mark Sisson, Robb Wolf, and others.

4. **FODMAPs**, which eliminates foods containing fructose, oligosaccharides, disaccharides, monosaccharides, alcohols, and polyols. These short chain carbs are known to cause stomach problems.

5. **Low-fat vegan diets**, which avoid "feeding" biofilms.

6. **Autoimmune and antihistamine diets**, which avoid common allergies like peanuts, soy, egg whites, and wheat.

7. **Dr. Kharrazian's and Dr. Lam's adrenal fatigue diets**, which are high in protein and low in carbs and gluten.

8. **Intermittent fasting**, which is used to metabolize accumulating pathogens and allow digestive rest.

9. **The Warrior Diet**, which suggests eating one massive meal at night while your parasympathetic nervous system (resting and digesting) is active, and fasting during the day when your sympathetic nervous system should be active (not resting and digesting, but fighting or "flighting").

10. **Dr. Wilson's fast and slow oxidizer diets**, which recommend different dietary choices based on your personal mineral ratios and oxidization pathways.

11. **The Wahls Diet**, which aims to support mitochondrial function by stuffing yourself with nine cups of vegetables a day.

12. **Ketogenic diets**, which remove all carbs from your diet in order to put you in a fasted state without fasting.

13.   **The Perfect Health Diet**, which eliminates grains, industrial oils, sugar and legumes.

14.   **Ray Peat's diet**, which eliminates grains, industrial oils and legumes but encourages sugar and fruit as sources of metabolic fuel.

Deep breath

With Lyme disease, things like collagen, magnesium, fat and sugar should be eliminated because they feed bacteria and biofilm. Or should these be increased, so we can make our bacteria and our bodies happy? With Lyme disease, eating a lot of vegetables can help us get the needed nutrients to protect our mitochondria and reduce MS- and ALS-type symptoms. Or do too many vegetables have goitrogenic effects and suppress our endocrine systems thus eventually hurting our mitochondria?

In excess, all food is poison. I say don't be a purist. Instead, be your own open-minded guinea pig to find out what works best for you.

CHAPTER 6: DIET TIPS

Lyme Diet Tips Experts *Actually* Agree On

If diet fads were countries they would all be at war. Diet is just one of those things on which we will never all agree. But there are some commonalities across these clashing schools of thought. This chapter will address eleven of these points of agreement. These aren't your typical diet tips, but the information here may give you guidance while you customize your own diet.

1.   Genetics Must Be Taken Into Account:

- Some ethnicities produce more of the enzyme amylase that breaks down carbs, making starches easier to digest, while some individuals have HLA gene mutations that affect starch and gluten digestion negatively.

- Some individuals have difficulty metabolising fructose, while others have difficulty metabolizing protein.

- While I advocate a moderate intake of saturated fats for most people, those with the Apolipoprotein E (APOE) gene (known as the Alzheimer's gene) do better with limited quantities.

- Many Lyme patients have MTHFR homozygous or heterozygous genes, which make methylation more difficult. This means taking synthetic B-vitamins is a big NO-NO and keeping an eye on your homocysteine levels can make a huge difference in your recovery.

- A genetic test can help you understand your personal epigenetics.

2.   Fermentable Carbs Feed Gut Bacteria

- Fiber ferments in our guts and feeds bacteria. Whether this is good or bad is widely disputed.

- I don't know if resistant starch feeds the "good" stuff or "bad" stuff.   However, resistant starch is best avoided, if you have Klebsiella in particular.

- I don't know if prebiotics like inulin and FOS are good or detrimental. Studies support both claims. I think it really depends on the individual.

- I also don't know if fiber is estrogenic as some experts claim, or anti-estrogenic because of its sweeping abilities.

3.   We Have More Research To Do On Probiotics

- Some studies suggest that probiotics prevent C. difficile; some studies suggest that they create endotoxins. Yet other studies suggest that some of the strains of our probiotics are actually "bad" bacteria.

- Some research supports that the gut should be sterile, meaning that fermented foods and non-enteric coated probiotics could worsen our conditions. Other research compares "germ free" rats to normal rats to see how they differ; the germ free rats are fatter and have weaker immune systems. This would suggest that the four pounds of gut bacteria (microbiome) we lug around help metabolize antigens, keep us lean, and support healthy immunity. Because I've experienced gut hell from antibiotic use (clindamycin, now THAT was a mistake), I have a biased leaning toward the latter argument.

- Check out brand reviews online before spending your money on a specific probiotic.

4. Getting Your Nutrition Through Food Is Superior to Getting It From Supplements

- Terry Wahls, author of *Minding My Mitochondria*, was right about at least one thing: synthetic vitamins don't support our bodies nearly as well as food. If you are deficient in something, google food sources and then decide whether or not these foods are appropriate for you and will cover the daily values you need. Some things, like vitamin D and magnesium, are hard to get through food alone. Supplementing with these might help, but I don't know for sure if these synthetic sources are good or harmful (studies both back and reject vitamin D, and some studies suggest we need magnesium supplementation while others suggest that magnesium feeds bacterial spirochetes).

- Make your diet nutrient dense, but consider extra supplementation if you are severely deficient or have genetic mutations to support.

5. **Sick People Should "Add" More Than They Should "Subtract"**

- This is something I hear Chinese medicine specialists say. Instead of restricting calories, patients should increase them. Instead of reducing body temperature with "cooling" foods, patients should increase body temperature with "warming foods". Fasting, chelation, and anything that, in one way or another, takes away something from your body will tax a weak body, no matter how miraculous the outcome may be. (That is not to say being aggressive about treatments is a bad thing.)

- I don't know if there is a time and place for fasting when sick, but even though fasting depletes adrenals, nutrients, and other body essentials, many people still vouch for fasting as a healing practice, believing it may increase the metabolism of pathogens.

- A note on fasting: When you initially reduce calories, your body goes through an anti-catabolic phase, where your body tissue is prevented from breaking down. Your metabolism gradually compensates by using metabolically active tissue as energy – namely muscle fiber. Muscle tissue is catabolized in a process of deamination – surrendering intramuscular branched chain amino acids (BCAAs) for use as energy. If you eat less over a long period, you will burn less. Your body adapts by *slowing* your metabolism. While slowing the metabolism, your body signals your thyroid, leptin and other hormones, telling the metabolism to use less and less energy. Because lean tissue sacrifices BCAAs for energy use, your body goes into "hoarding mode," so that it uses calories for storage and not to build lean tissue. Just keep this in mind before doing an extended fast.

6. Herxing Should Be Temporary

- In my opinion, extreme herxing (feeling crummy due to the "die off" of an infection) is not a sign of good things to come. A mild herx is okay, but a severe herx may actually slow your recovery.

- If your lymph glands are swollen, slow down on the bug-killing. Swollen lymph glands may mean that you are not eliminating antigens (possibly dead-bug debris) fast enough to keep up with the pace at which you are killing them.

- If a herx is lasting days or weeks without improvement, it may not be a herx at all. Rather, you may be experiencing drug side effects from a poor xenobiotic metabolism, something we will talk more about in Chapter 8.

7. We Are Confused About Omega 6 Ratios

- Most experts agree that we need a balanced ratio of omega 3 to 6, but they do not all agree on what that ratio is and which foods to get them from.

- Minimizing omega 6 might be a better option than mega-dosing on fish oil (omega 3) to balance out exceedingly high omega 6 levels. This is not to say that you should remove nuts and seeds from your diet. But perhaps, if your intention of supplementing with fish oil is to trump omega 6 ratios in your body, consider instead reducing the amount of industrial oils you use in your diet, as these are high in omega 6 fats.

- When it comes to omega 6 rich foods, fresh sources are significantly healthier. For example, eat your nuts out of their shells or your egg yolks soon after cracking your eggs. The longer these sit out, the more oxidative damage they incur.

- Some omega 6 rich foods are particularly high in aflatoxins, a toxin produced by mold that some people are sensitive to. These include peanuts and Brazil nuts.

8. Just Because We Are Told Something Is Good for Us Does Not Mean That It Is

- It's easy to get caught up in one perspective when there is a lot of info out there that supports it. But question everything – especially if you are overly gung-ho about it. Doubt what you read and what your doctor tells you. Have patience and research contradictory theories before you go popping every pill an expert tells you to take.

- Some diet tips are good for one group of people but bad for others. For example, I cannot suggest we all chow down on calf liver, because some genetic mutations make metabolising organ meats really hard. I cannot suggest that we all eat low-carb high-fat diets, because this would hurt a lot of people. Those who weight train need more carbs than sedentary people. Spirochetes rob us of our sugars, but I cannot suggest that we eliminate sugars to stop feeding them *nor* can I suggest we increase our sugar intake so that we have sugars for ourselves, too. I cannot suggest that we all eat meat. Those who are frail and pale tend to do better with meat in their diets, but some people really do better on vegetarian diets. Hell, I've seen vegan bodybuilders, though I have no clue how they pull it off!

- Balance is key. For instance, your Th-1 and Th-2 cells should be in balance; you should not be too hot or too cold; your urine should not be too clear or too yellow; your pulse should not be too high or too low; we should not exercise too much or allow physical deconditioning…you get the point.

- Here's something that took me a long time to learn: too much of a good thing ain't a good thing. I'm talking about F.O.O.D.

- I have tried juice fasting, eating meat 3 times a day, eating heaps of saturated fat all day, going vegan, doing paleo, trying other diets like the SCD, Wahls, and GAPS diets; golly, I've tried just about every fad diet out there. I was disciplined with each one, too (you can ask my mom). I lost my healthy relationship with food and started viewing it as either medicine or poison. The fact is *it is all poison* when you eat too much of it.

- Finally, I don't know what your balance will be compared to mine, but I do know it would be nice if you found it!

9. What You Eat Really Can Affect Your Hormones

- Like medications, what you eat has the ability to produce unwanted side effects.

- Some foods, like flax and soy, have phytoestrogens, which affect estrogen production. Whether they increase or decrease estrogen levels in the body is still up for debate.

- Some foods are high in polyunsaturated fats, which some doctors suggest suppress thyroid function. I avoid eating excess PUFA's but others swear by their nuts and seeds. Soaking, sprouting and cooking foods high in these gets rid of some of the phytic acid that comes in the PUFA-package. Phytic acid is claimed by some to be an "anti-nutrient" and others to be an "anti-oxidant." I gather it is a bit of both.

- Goitrogenic foods may suppress thyroid function, but I don't think they are the cause of hypothyroidism. The brassica family is especially goitrogenic. This means broccoli, cabbage, spinach and kale *may* not be as good for you as you previously thought. Cooking them in water removes some goitrogens.

- Gliadin can allegedly be absorbed from a leaky gut into the bloodstream. It should not be there thus the body produces an immune response to target and destroy (metabolize) it. The gliadin compound in gluten also shares a similar-looking molecular structure to our thyroid hormones. Can our bodies mistake our thyroid hormones for gliadin molecules and attack them as well? It depends who you ask. Either way, if you feel fine when you eat gluten, don't let the GF Nazis scare you.

10. Some Foods Make Biofilm, Heavy Metals, and Infections Worse

- I can see why low-fat diets work, because fat may increase biofilm. But carbs can feed bacteria, and fish are high in mercury. So…should we just eat red meat, drink water and call it a day? Like I said, all food is poison in high quantities.

- Biofilm may require fat, but without some fat in our diets our hormones suffer and our joints start to hurt (every time I've tried going VLC, my hips hurt within 24 hours).

- Bacteria may utilize sugar, but without carbs our glycogen stores deplete and our bodies look for fuel elsewhere. This usually means they catabolize body tissue into glucose so it can be used as fuel. Although I am *so* guilty for fearing dem' sugar-eating buggers, some studies suggest that if we completely remove sugars from our diets, the bacteria in our guts will look elsewhere for fuel and thus burrow into our gut linings. Not to mention, if we remove carbs from our diets completely, the "good" bacteria die, too. Other studies suggest that sugar – when taken in conjunction with antibiotics – actually acts like bait to draw persister bacteria out of hiding.

11. Infections Leach Nutrients From Our Bodies

- Iron, collagen, sugar, calcium, magnesium, manganese…these are just some of the things that spirochetes feed on or use as building blocks for biofilm. I can tell you that much. But I can't tell you whether you should avoid these so that you end up losing some battles but winning the war. Neither can I advise you to increase them so that you don't end up magnesium deficient and having seizures, or collagen deficient and having heart attacks. Everything feeds bacteria. Personally, I avoid foods that make me feel inflamed but I don't avoid "bug-foods." I feel like I need to have enough magnesium and sugar for them *and* for me. No more, no less. That said, I am also at a point in my treatment where I have greatly reduced my infectious load, at least to the point where my symptoms are minimal.

- Now this is the million-dollar question: With Lyme disease, should collagen, magnesium, fat and sugar be eliminated because they feed bacteria and biofilm, or should they be increased, so we can support our "good" bacteria and keep our bodies happy? Contact me at yessington@itsnotjustlyme.com if you would like to share your thoughts on this dilemma.

CHAPTER 7: LYME AND CALORIES

Do Sick People Need More or Fewer Calories?

Based on my research and personal experience, I've found that illness is associated with an increased resting energy expenditure, which means chronically ill patients actually need *more calories.*

When you are *chronically* sick, your metabolism gets worn out. For every degree colder your body gets, your metabolism gets slower.

But if sick people have sloppy metabolisms, does that mean they should be fasting and keeping their calories to a minimum?

Nope. First of all, if you don't eat adequate calories, your body assumes food is scarce and your metabolism slows further. Secondly, if you are not dead yet it means your body is fighting. Fighting takes *a lot of energy.*

This means that if you are lying in bed *with* a cold, you burn more calories than you would lying in bed *without* a cold.

Metabolic interventionist, Dr. Rifka Schulman, has gathered research based on decades of experience with critical care patients. The goal of metabolic intervention is to provide adequate nutrition in near-perfect ratios of macronutrients (carbs, proteins, fats) and to ensure body systems maintain function in times of critical care.

Over decades of metabolic intervention with CCI patients, here is what has been gathered:

- Providing adequate nutrition early on can assist immune and catabolic responses, preserve gastrointestinal integrity and support healing.

- Underfeeding and overfeeding are equally detrimental, but underfeeding is more common.

Let's take a look at how underfeeding can affect ill patients. Underfeeding proteins, carbs and fats each have distinguishable outcomes:

- Protein deficiencies can slow healing, increase infections, cause muscle wasting, and deplete diaphragmatic muscles.

- Low-carb, high-fat diets may cause delayed gastric emptying. Carb deficiencies are particularly devastating to the endocrine system and the metabolism.

- Fat deficiencies deprive us of a transport system for fat-soluble vitamins and of the precursors to cortisol and sex hormones.

***Let Me Just Say*, "I Think Lyme Disease Patients Are Generally Underfed."**

We have so many dietary restrictions (and fears) that we often don't meet our own caloric needs. This slows down our metabolisms even further, and it becomes increasingly uncomfortable to eat much at all.

We are also told to cut back on carbs, so a lot of us have developed a fear of sugar. Sugar may feed bacteria, but so do essential amino acids and minerals. If we stop ingesting amino acids, certain necessary bodily processes will not happen. Likewise, if we stop eating carbs, essential metabolic processes slow down.

I for one would rather catabolize carbs for energy than have my own muscles break down for energy. I'd rather have my body *and* the critters well fed than have my body start eating itself.

(P.S.: Our stomachs have immune cells that can be disrupted with starvation, allowing antigens to leak into our circulatory systems. This is one reason underfeeding is linked to increased infections. Makes me think twice about fasting, which may force the critters to bite holes in my stomach lining in their desperation to survive.)

BUT (and there is always a *but*) adding calories too quickly can also be detrimental. What's more, some people are overfeeding and actually *do* need to cut back on calories.

Refeeding Syndrome

Refeeding syndrome can occur when sick people start adding calories too quickly. It can cause electrolyte imbalances, along with a whole array of hematological problems.

Dr. Schulman says it best:

"Starvation, with minimal or no carbohydrate intake, reduces insulin and increases glucagon levels. In the absence of insulin, metabolic pathways shift to promote lipolysis, free fatty acid oxidation, and ketone production for energy. With the reintroduction of carbohydrates there is an increased demand for phosphorylated intermediates of glycolysis (adenosine triphosphate [ATP] and 2,3-diphosphoglycerate [2,3-DPG]), depleting phosphate stores, which are already low due to poor nutrition and usually vitamin D deficiency. A surge in insulin secretion in response to carbohydrate load shifts phosphorus, potassium, and magnesium into cells, lowering serum levels further, and has a renal anti-natriuretic effect, with resultant sodium and water retention. Demand for thiamine is raised as well, predisposing to deficiency and associated complications. Other micronutrients are abnormally redistributed as well in the refeeding syndrome. Severe hypophosphatemia can impair diaphragmatic function and impede weaning from the ventilator."

For these reasons, refeeding syndrome can make chronically ill people sicker when they add calories too quickly. If refeeding syndrome is suspected, limit carbs until phosphate levels have stabilized. Vitamin D should be raised in cases of hypophosphatemia. Increase calories in small increments (i.e. 200 calorie per day increments).

For the Overfed

Overfeeding can be just as harmful as caloric restriction. In general it's linked to increased infection and liver dysfunction.

Specifically:

- Carb overfeeding can impair glycemic control.

- Lipid overfeeding can increase inflammation through the production of inflammatory eicosanoids (eicosanoids are derived from fatty acids and can be pro- or anti-inflammatory).

- Last but not least, protein overfeeding can increase ammonia levels, oxidative deamination and dehydration.

Who Should Reduce Caloric Intake?

Certain drugs and conditions reduce energy needs. In terms of drugs, sedatives, analgesics and neuromuscular blocking agents reduce resting energy expenditure.

In terms of conditions, obesity complicates resting energy expenditure. Excess fat lowers metabolism because adipose tissue is storage tissue with a lower metabolic activity. Also, fat is almost *too good* at storing energy, so it doesn't need to be burned as much. This means our metabolism slows down when we are overweight, simply because it can.

Pay attention to signs of overfeeding. Measure BUN levels to determine if protein intake should be reduced. Dr. Schulman suggests "Clinically important elevations in BUN (> 70 mg/dL) or ammonia (> 70 μg/dL) should prompt a reduction of protein and/or increase in hydration." Conversely, if you have hyperglycemia, consider reducing non-protein calories.

Okay, so how do you know if you are underfed or overfed?

Calculate REE to Determine How Many Calories You Need

Your resting energy expenditure (REE) is the minimum amount of calories you need when you are sedentary in order to fuel your body without leaching energy from your muscles. The REE is higher in chronically sick people because their bodies are constantly fighting. So the sicker you are, the more calories you burn just sitting on your ass. Winning!

A simple formula recommended by the American College of Chest Physicians' 1997 consensus statement is to take 25 calories for every kilogram of body weight, to avoid both overfeeding and underfeeding.

Another formula presented by the American Dietetic Association is a little more complicated:

For men REE is calculated with this formula:

$10 \times \text{weight (kg)} + 6.25 \times \text{height (cm)} - 5 \times \text{age (y)} + 5$

For women REE is calculated with this formula:

$10 \times \text{weight (kg)} + 6.25 \times \text{height (cm)} - 5 \times \text{age (y)} - 161.$

There are other equations that require your fat free mass, and yet others that require your oxygen input and output. Keep in mind that these equations are theoretical and only estimate the bare minimum needed to survive. Take for instance the first formula I mentioned – this represents the amount of calories used in feeding tubes for patients in comas. Needless to say, you need more calories than that to move and go about your daily life. These formulas put me at around 1200 to 1300 calories a day, but I don't spend my waking hours in bed so I typically eat over double of that in a day. I'll rest when I'm dead, yo (totally joking; I <3 couches).

You typically need around 1-2 grams of protein per kilogram of body weight and you can get the rest of your calories from carbs and fats. The more energy you expend, the more carbs you need. And remember, if you are ill then the amount of calories you need goes up. Extremely sedentary people *may* do better with high-fat low-carb diets, but too few carbs causes hormonal problems. I do best with a diet of 45% carbs, 35% proteins and 20% fats, but this takes into account 5 days a week of anaerobic exercise. If I were sedentary, my protein intake would remain the same, but I would increase fats and decrease carbs in my diet.

There is no one perfect equation for caloric intake and macronutrient ratios for chronically ill people (or healthy people for that matter). All we know is that age, sex, presence of fever or inflammation, thyroid function, and so much more can influence REE.

Like all things Lyme, you really need to experiment to find out what works.

In Summary

- Underfeeding and overfeeding work against chronically ill patients.

- Either of these can increase infections, so avoid starvation and binging.

- If you are underfed, eat more calories to give your body the hint to speed up your metabolic rate to burn your fuel. The more fuel you have, the easier it is to burn that fuel.

- If you are overfed, determine if you should reduce protein, carbs, or fats.

Enjoy your food. You're probably going to need a lot more of it!

CHAPTER 8: DRUG METABOLISM

Most people are not experts on drug metabolism, but I think we can all agree that drugs are frakkin awesome! They make us trip out and see unicorns, they make pain seemingly vanish, or they make us so incredibly happy that we never want to be without them again. Quoting Louis C.K., "drugs are so f***ing good they'll ruin your life."

Given that many people with Lyme have throbbing and sharp full-body pains, inflammation, adrenal deficiency, depression, and other pains, drugs can be literal life-savers. Nonetheless, despite their fantastic individual effects, being on more than one drug at a time can create adverse reactions.

What Is Drug Metabolism?

Drug metabolism happens when your body changes drugs, or xenobiotics, into more easily excreted products with the help of special enzymes. In other words, it prevents drugs from accumulating in your body by detoxifying them out. Yes, detoxification was a scientific *thing* before the alternative medicine hippies branded the word.

How It Works

Metabolising drugs takes a lot of effort. Generally, xenobiotics cannot be excreted in the urine until they have undergone a process to make them soluble in water. Drug metabolism usually occurs in the liver, which houses the enzymes needed to metabolize the drugs.

There are 2 phases of metabolism. Some drugs undergo both phases, while other drugs only undergo one of them:

Phase 1 metabolism is when the cytochrome P450 (CYP450) enzymes in the liver oxidize drugs. This makes them smaller and thus easier to excrete from the body.

Phase 2 metabolism is when an ionised group attaches to a drug. These groups include glutathione, methyl or acetyl groups. They make the drug more water soluble and thus easier to excrete.

Overdose

When a drug has accumulated beyond your body's detoxifying capacities, it can cause toxicity or hepatitis. This can occur when there is not enough glutathione to detoxify the drug out of your body. NAC (a precursor to glutathione) is actually quite the popular supplement in the rave community – a community that surely OD's a lot.

Taking glutathione can help metabolize drugs and save your liver, but it will also remove the drugs from your body quicker. (Hmmm, why not just take less of the drugs so you don't tax your liver in the first place and so you don't waste your money on supplements to counteract your drugs? Sorry to go off topic but *ugh*, this is all too frustratingly common.)

Inducers, Inhibitors and Adverse Reactions

Inhibitors are drugs that stop enzymes from working as effectively. In other words, a drug that inhibits enzymes from metabolising it makes it (along with whatever other drugs you are taking) stay in the body longer.

Inducers make enzymes work better. So essentially, an inducer drug has the opposite effect of an inhibitor and speeds up the process of moving it (and whatever other drugs you are taking) out of the body quicker.

In this sense, when you are taking a medication, you are not just taking a drug – you are also taking either an inhibitor or an inducer. Adverse drug reactions can occur because of this. Let's say you take the antibiotic Erythromycin (an inhibitor), and you also like to drink grapefruit juice everyday (also an inhibitor). As a result, last night's dose of antibiotics might stagnate in your liver longer than expected. This is bad news if you're ready to pop your next dose. If you don't have enough glutathione (or other detoxifying agents) to compensate for an overload of Erythromycin in your body, a toxic overdose or liver damage can occur.

Other Factors

Sex, age, and even gut bacteria composition affect drug metabolism. Genetic deficiencies of particular enzymes can play a big role as well. For example, some people suck at metabolising codeine, while others metabolize it quickly. A small dose of codeine could kill a slow metabolizer, but do nothing for a quick one.

Even the food you eat is a factor in how drugs are metabolized! As I mentioned, grapefruit juice is an inhibitor. So is pomegranate. Brussels sprouts and garlic, on the other hand, are inducers.

Here's just one more to blow your mind: cigarette smoke is also an inducer.

In Summary

When CYP450 enzymes are inhibited or induced by drugs, clinically significant drug-to-drug interactions can cause adverse reactions. Knowing which ones inhibit and which ones induce your enzymes can minimize the possibility of negative interactions between all those pills you pop to (try to) feel normal. If they are not doing what they are supposed to – or if you think you are having a month long herx – then you may be having an adverse drug reaction.

CHAPTER 9: NUTRIENTS LEACHED BY INFECTIONS AND DRUGS

Recall that metabolism is the body's way of breaking down and building up energy at a cellular level. Without this process, the vitamins and minerals we eat and produce inside of us would not be used effectively. Fighting any illness, whether affecting cardiovascular, immune, hematological, neurological, viral or hormonal systems, requires nutrients that can only be made useful by proper metabolism. Nutrient metabolism has endless benefits:

- Nutrients are needed to produce neurotransmitters and hormones.

- Vitamins and minerals help convert nutrients and are needed for continued metabolic health.

- Fatty acids form the structures of our cells.

- Flavonoids and carotenoids help cells function.

- Vitamins, minerals and other nutrients are all needed to build muscle. Stronger muscles correlate with stronger metabolisms.

- Many more, and *this* is why we ought to take nutrient depletions seriously.

  Now let's take a look at what depletes what.

Infections Can Deplete Nutrients

As mentioned in Chapter 2:

- Mycoplasma depends on inflammation and immune dysregulation to thrive.

- Babesia and Bartonella depend on inflammation and immune dysregulation to infect red blood cells.

- Ehrlichia and Anaplasma depend on inflammation and immune dysregulation to infect white blood cells.

- Lyme disease depends on inflammation to deteriorate collagen into bug meal.

- And the list goes on.

Drugs Can Deplete Nutrients

Here are some of the deficiencies, as described by James LaValle in *Cracking the Metabolic Code,* which can occur when taking the following common prescription drugs:

Deficiencies Due to the Antibiotics Known as Penicillins, Cephalosporins, Fluoroquinolones, Macrolides and Aminoglycosides:

- Biotin

- Inositol

- Lactobacillus acidophilus

- Bifidobacteria bifidum

- B1

- B2

- B3

- B6

- B12

- Vitamin K

Deficiencies Due to the Antibiotics Known as Tetracyclines and Sulfonamides:

- Biotin

- Calcium

- Inositol

- Iron

- Lactobacillus acidophilus

- Bifidobacteria bifidum

- Magnesium

- B1

- B2

- B3

- B6

- B12

- Vitamin K

Deficiencies Due to the Antibiotic Neomycin:

- Beta carotene

- Iron

- Vitamin A

- Vitamin B12

Deficiencies Due to the Antibiotic Co-Trimoxazole:

- Lactobacillus acidophilus

- Bifidobacteria bifidus

- Folic acid

Deficiencies Due to the Antibiotic Isoniazid:

- B3

- B6

- Vitamin D

Deficiencies Due to the Antibiotic Rifampin:

- Vitamin D

Deficiencies Due to the Antibiotic Ethambutol:

- Copper

- Zinc

Deficiencies Due to Salicylates:

- Folic acid

- Iron

- Potassium

- Sodium

- Vitamin C

Deficiencies Due to NSAIDs:

- Folic acid

Deficiencies Due to Corticosteroids:

- Calcium

- Folic acid

- Magnesium

- Potassium

- Selenium

- Vitamin C

- Vitamin D

- Zinc

Deficiencies Due to Reverse Transcription Inhibitors and Non-Nucleosides:

- Carnitine

- Copper

- B12

- Zinc

Deficiencies Due to Cholestyramine:

- Beta carotene

- Calcium

- Folic acid

- Iron

- Magnesium

- Phosphorus

- Vitamin A

- B12

- Vitamin D

- Vitamin K

- Vitamin E

- Zinc

These drugs and infections in the body can greatly tax the liver. A lot of doctors recommend taking anti-oxidants to off-set this effect. Glutathione is known for its liver detoxifying effects in the Lyme world, but I have some thoughts on why we may be over doing glutathione.

First, a Note on Antioxidants

Oxidation occurs when electrons are pulled from substances, creating reactive substances or "free radicals." Conversely, *antioxidants* prevent oxidation, and thus reduce tissue damage. But too many anti-oxidants can interfere with healthy oxidation. Despite popular belief, some oxidation is a good thing.

Our cells need oxygen. Not too much, not too little. Oxygen can kill bacteria. That's why your doctor tells you to let cuts n' scrapes "breathe" and why oxidative substances like hydrogen peroxide kill germs on contact. Hydrogen peroxide is also generated within your body in order to kill internal germs. Also, when combined with iodine in your body, hydrogen is highly oxidative, which leads to the necessary production of thyroid hormones. See, oxidation is not all that bad.

So, anti-oxidants are good. But too many can interfere with healthy oxidation. Oxidation is good, but too much oxidation can cause tissue damage.

Now, Some Thoughts on Glutathione and NAC

Liposomal-, IV- and even suppository-glutathione have become popular treatments in the Lyme community. Glutathione, an anti-oxidant made from 3 amino acids (glutamine, cysteine, and glycine) has been dubbed the "Mother of all antioxidants" and rightfully so. People claim to stand up out of their wheelchairs for 30 minutes following IV glutathione sessions, as it dramatically and quickly detoxifies their livers.

For a quick fix, supplementing with glutathione or its precursor NAC can sometimes help. After a night of tequila shots or a bout of acute acetaminophen poisoning,

NAC is really awesome to have in your medicine cabinet. It's also a good addition if you are methionine deficient.

But as a daily supplement, I am on the fence. I stopped taking NAC orally and glutathione intravenously after I read Joey Lott's *The Mother of All Antioxidants*. I felt okay when I took these on a weekly basis but I didn't feel any worse once I stopped. Nor did I go into remission until I stopped (though I do not think they prevented my recovery).

Yes, we probably are low in glutathione when fighting chronic infections, so I don't think a little bit will hurt. But supplementing with 1000mg a day of NAC might be overkill. Glutathione can reduce oxidation so much so that those dang bugs you want dead will thank you (remember, oxidation kills germs). It can also quickly remove the medications from your body that, unlike tequila, you do *not* want detoxed immediately.

Natural Solutions

Instead of supplementing daily with glutathione and NAC, support healthy glutathione production naturally with foods that contain the nutrients below:

- Glycine, which helps convert homocysteine into cysteine (one of the 3 amino acids that make glutathione).

- Betaine, B12, B6, and folate also help, although too much of these can cause over-methylation.

- Protein aids in glutathione production.

- Molybdenum reduces homocysteine.

- Remember, if you "need" extra glutathione because you are overdosing on antibiotics, what you might actually need is a lower dose of antibiotics.

CHAPTER 10: EXERCISE AND MITOCHONDRIA

We all know that exercise *can* be beneficial when done properly. In this final chapter, I will address how exercise works, why it matters for Lyme recovery, and the limitations of exercising due to physical pain.

How Exercise Works

Remember when we talked about how ATP is used by our cells as energy? Well, ATP is also imperative for exercise. The energy from ATP helps muscles contract during exercise. We constantly create more ATP during exercise, whether our exercise is aerobic (using oxygen) or anaerobic (without using oxygen).

Carbs are the main energy source for high intensity exercise, whereas fats are helpful for low intensity exercise. Proteins typically maintain and repair muscles afterwards, but are not used to fuel workouts.

Muscles have a few seconds worth of ATP in them for you to start sprinting without oxygen. After that, you can sprint for another couple seconds by converting the creatine phosphate in your muscles into ATP. Once you run out of creatine phosphate, you start metabolising carbs to create more ATP. A high intensity exercise can produce twenty times more ATP when there is oxygen involved (basically, once you start breathing heavily).

You can exercise for hours at a low intensity, because aerobic exercise is fueled by fat (and fat is stored in abundance). However, this type of exercise does not tend to help you build muscle.

In short, the more a muscle works, the more it metabolizes ATP. The more ATP you lose, the more ATP your body creates to replace it.

Why It Matters

Consider the following:

- Your mitochondria produce ATP.

- ATP gives you energy.

- Your muscles are loaded with mitochondria.

- The more muscle you have, the more mitochondria you have.

- The more mitochondria you have, the more ATP you can produce and burn to fuel your cells.

Muscles are loaded with mitochondria to provide huge quantities of ATP for them so that you can, among other things, pick your ass up off the couch.

Forty years ago Professor John Holloszy of Washington U found that exercise produced an increase in muscular mitochondria, as well as an increase in the uptake of glucose from the blood into the muscles (this point, in particular, is significant for those who fear that glucose feeds their hematological infections).

Basically, your body recognizes your demand for more energy when you exercise. So ATP production increases as you use your muscles by producing more mitochondria. In turn, more mitochondria = more ATP production.

Use It or Lose It

If you don't use your muscles, you can lose mitochondrial content. A decline in mitochondria makes us age faster and correlates with countless illnesses, particularly degenerative illnesses like MS, Alzheimer's, Parkinson's, diabetes, and heart disease. Without these powerhouses up and running, we stop effectively turning our food into fuel for our cells. Without this fuel, fighting a chronic infection can become a bigger challenge than it already is.

Hey look at that; we've come full circle! I guess it's time to end this book. But first, I want to tell you a story about my grandpa, Big Sam.

Don't Let Pain Stop You

Big Sam was a toy salesman, a philanthropist, and a charismatic and totally offensive comic. He looked like Bob Barker, with the white hair, deep tan, baby-coloured golf shirts, and tall lanky build. In his eighties, he developed aphasia and slowly lost his ability to speak. Once upon a time he was a big talker, but eventually our conversations started to go like this:

> Me: Hi grandpa!
>
> Big Sam: Ya!
>
> Me: How are you?
>
> Big Sam: Ya! Ya?
>
> Me: I'm good, thanks!

Imagine making a living with your mouth, only to have your words taken away. Anyways, he also took prednisone for bullous pemphigoid (some rare autoimmune condition that manifested in his seventies), which gave him burning neuropathy in his feet. Now imagine being an avid athlete and a healthy eater into your seventies and suddenly finding your body deteriorating from the feet up and the head down.

Why am I telling you this? Basically I am just trying to explain that I watched someone lose his speech, a characteristic that defined his whole life. He adapted his epic jokes first into one liners, then into one-worders, and finally, just into big smiles. I've watched an almost-ninety year old dude in excruciating pain - unable to walk much because of his burning feet - get in and out of a pool to swim laps (mind you, at a turtle-pace). After one episode in the hospital (where my whole family went to say "goodbye" but he miraculously recovered) he knew his swimming days were over. Still, he made sure to get up once an hour to walk around the house for two minutes or so just to keep things flowing.

Big Sam lived longer than many people expected. At his funeral, if anyone told my grandma "he's in peace now", she would bark at them, "He was in peace while he was alive!" Even though some people wouldn't consider it "much of a life", he preferred the combo of pain and laughter to giving up and deteriorating even more rapidly.

I'm not trying to undermine your pain by any means. I'm just saying that as valid of an excuse as pain is to put off exercising, there are ways of accommodating your illness. I mean, squeeze your butt cheeks together really tight in your wheelchair if that is what it takes! Pushing yourself for even two-minutes of exercise a day can improve your mitochondrial content and your energy production. Try it and you might even impress yourself.

CONCLUSION

Funny enough, this all started with a tablespoon of honey. It made me question my notion that carbs were my enemy and helped me get to where I am today. I feel healthy and I plan to continue feeling healthy. (Although if things change, I will let you know.) But my fight for remission goes beyond diet; it goes beyond exercising; it goes beyond supporting my endocrine system, adrenals, reproductive system, liver and genetics. There is always more to the puzzle.

This book captures only a small piece of the puzzle. Nonetheless, here is a summary of what was addressed above.

In Summary

Metabolism is the breakdown and build-up of all sorts of things such as micronutrients, macronutrients, drugs, muscles, and ATP. Lyme slows metabolism because it is a chronic stressor. Also, a slow metabolism slows recovery because it starves our cells of energy.

A good metabolism correlates with better gastrin production and thus food digestion. Better digestion means more nutrients for your cells. The thyroid works better when your cells are nourished and in consequence so does your liver. A healthy liver helps you convert T4 into T3, allows you to eliminate excess estrogen and detoxifies xenobiotics. A healthy metabolism will also increase your body temperature, which warms you and increases enzymatic processes that are helpful in metabolising both drugs and food. Increasing your metabolism overall boosts immunity, protects red blood cells and inhibits inflammation. It energizes and optimizes us.

Chronic stress is the beginning of the end for metabolic health. Once your body starts neglecting the production of sex hormones in favor of extra cortisol, the adrenals, your sex hormones and your thyroid lose their synergistic balance.

Hypothyroidism is bad news, but all too common for Lyme patients. A healthy thyroid, on the other hand, is good for GI and liver function, growth hormone production, burning fat, metabolising glucose, regulating cholesterol and sex hormones, and fixing anemia. Some foods and herbs are more supportive for thyroid function than others, so educate yourself on what is supportive to the thyroid and what is goitrogenic.

Question everything you've ever believed about the perfect diet (or Lyme protocol for that matter); there's no such thing. I was careful not to make many foodie suggestions because there are too many individual factors to consider that, frankly, I don't know about you. That said, you can check out my own dietary and supplementary protocol on itsnotjustlyme.com for some ideas.

If you eat or take anything because you believe it is healthy, yet you've been "herxing" for months, please re-evaluate. Everything you put into your body is metabolized. Some of those substances can induce or inhibit your CYP450 enzymes, so keep in mind that adverse reactions can occur between multiple drugs and even between drugs and what you eat.

Bacteria can feed on glucose, magnesium, iron, fat, collagen, amino acids, you name it! I don't think we should eliminate these from our diets, because they feed us, too. Underfeeding fats, for example, can deprive us of a transport system for fat soluble vitamins. Meanwhile, high-fat, low-carb diets can cause delayed gastric emptying. Carb deficiencies are particularly devastating to your metabolism. I think most Lyme patients are underfed, although overfeeding can also backfire. It's cliché but balance is key. You can calculate your resting energy expenditure to determine the minimum amount of calories you need at rest.

Another good reason to eat carbs is to fuel exercise. As daunting as exercise can be, it builds muscle. The more muscle you build, the more loaded with mitochondria your muscles become. Mitochondria produce ATP, which fuel your cells to undergo all the metabolic processes that keep you alive and strong. The more mitochondria you have, the quicker you can convert food into fuel, catabolize and anabolize, detoxify, and fight...anything. The fewer mitochondria you have, the more prone you are to ALS- and MS-type symptoms.

So, despite the pains involved in using and producing energy efficiently, despite the layered approaches that require trial and error to get it right, it's worth the trouble. I hope I have convinced you that a healthy metabolism is an essential part of getting to and staying in remission. I wanted this book to educate more than advise you, however I did mention a few applicable health strategies. A summary of these can be found in the next and final section.

REMEDIES

This is not a complete list of Lyme remedies, but rather suggestions that are specific to optimizing metabolism.

Adrenals, adaptogens for: Include ashwagandha, rhodiola and maca, among others. Research herbs before use. A 24 hour cortisol test can help determine if you are low or high in cortisol.

Adrenals, nutrients for: Vitamin C, Vitamin D, B-complex, and magnesium; food sources are best.

Breakfast: Restores liver glycogen; good for stress, adrenals and the endocrine system.

Calories: If you move, sit, stand, or do anything other than sleep, you need more calories than what is suggested by REE formulas. Try to eat 1-2 grams of protein per kilogram of body weight and get the rest from carbs and fats. Eat more carbs if you exercise and more fats if you are sedentary, but still ingest enough carbs that you do not deplete your glycogen stores.

Carbs: Give us glucose and energy for mitochondria. They are good for exercise and to stimulate the endocrine system. Carbs are not all created equally, but different theories support and oppose all of them, so experiment to see what works for you.

Diet: Don't join a diet cult; instead, find your ratio of macronutrients and micronutrients needed to improve your health and experiment with food from there.

Drug metabolism: Research which of your drugs are inducers and which are inhibitors. Avoid or minimize adverse drug reactions. Consider having a genetic test done. Also, consider supplementing nutrients that are leached from specific drugs (refer to Chapter 9 for specifics).

Exercise: Build muscle to replicate mitochondria. Consider using weight resistance exercises such as yoga or resistance training. Tai Chi is a low impact exercise that can be performed while seated. Consider adopting any exercise where you aren't out of breath for long periods. Try exercising for *at least* 2 minutes a day.

Fats: Turn into glycerol and fatty acids; these are good for hormone production and fat soluble vitamins. Try reducing your intake of polyunsaturated fats, especially those high in omega 6 and aflatoxins.

Fear of sugar: Try what I did – a tablespoon of honey in the morning when your glycogen is low, so the glucose uptake is quick. Also, if you take it away from food and drink it is absorbed higher up in the GI tract (avoiding the lower intestinal tract, where people tend to be concerned that sugars will feed infections). Try it for 3 days and see how you feel. Most likely, your body could use some extra carbs, and this is a good trick to get them.

Genetic testing: Helps determine what foods, vitamins, additives, xenobiotics and pollutants you have a hard time metabolising.

Glutathione: Increase this naturally by increasing glycine, betaine, B12, B6, folate, protein and molybdenum. Take NAC or glutathione occasionally or for drug induced "hangovers."

Liver function: A healthy liver is good for converting T4 to T3, for eliminating excess estrogen and to detoxify xenobiotics. Consider taking milk thistle. Also, try lightly pushing on your liver (or your right side) to move stagnation; this will either help you or do nothing.

Magnesium: This is good for sleep, stress and for promoting hundreds of enzymatic processes in your body. It may, however, feed certain infections.

Manuka honey: A good source of methylglyoxal and glucose.

Proteins: Proteins give us amino acids and synthesize into hemoglobin, hormones, enzymes, and plasma proteins. Try ingesting daily at least .8 grams of protein per kilogram of body weight and at most 2.4 grams per kilogram of body weight. Elevations in BUN (> 70 mg/dL) or ammonia (> 70 µg/dL) should prompt you to reduce protein intake and/or increase hydration.

Sleep: Ideally, go to sleep by 10pm. Magnesium and B6 can be helpful.

Stimulants: Limit them to low cortisol hours (9:30am to 11:30am and 3:30pm to 5:30pm).

Thyroid health: Eliminate gluten. Get adequate tyrosine, selenium and protein. Eat saturated fats, but limit polyunsaturated fats. Reduce goitrogenic foods and balance your hormones.

Thyroid, herbs that support: Nettle and guggul assist with T4 to T3 conversion; bacopa increases T4.

Thyroid, herbs that suppress: Japanese knotweed, isatis, sida acuta, valerian root, passionflower, motherwort and large doses of quercetin; possibly cannabis, green tea and curcumin.

WORKS CITED

This is a collection of textbooks, articles and books that influenced the making of this book. I've also included websites below, which I referenced in this book. If you believe everything you read, please don't read! Otherwise, these works can educate you further on the science and controversy regarding infections, metabolism, immunity, diet, and so forth.

Applegate, Edith J. *The Anatomy and Physiology Learning System*. St. Louis, MO: Saunders/Elsevier, 2011. Print.

Blaser, Martin J. *Missing Microbes: How the Overuse of Antibiotics Is Fueling Our Modern Plagues*. New York, NY: Henry Holt and Co., 2014. Print.

Bowthorpe, Janie A., and Paige Adams. *Stop the Thyroid Madness: How Thyroid Experts Are Challenging Ineffective Treatments and Improving the Lives of Patients*. Dolores, CO: Laughing Grape Pub., 2014. Print.

Buhner, Stephen. *Healing Lyme: Natural Prevention and Treatment of Lyme Borreliosis and Its Coinfections*. White River Junction, VT: Chelsea Green Publishing, 2005. Print.

Gibson, G. G., and Paul Skett. *Introduction to Drug Metabolism*. Cheltenham, UK: Nelson Thornes, 2001. Print.

Holloszy, John O., and Edward F. Coyle. "Adaptations of Skeletal Muscle to Endurance Exercise and Their Metabolic Consequences." *Journal of Applied Physiology* (1989): *National Center for Biotechnology Information*. U.S. National Library of Medicine. Web.

Horowitz, Richard I. *Why Can't I Get Better? Solving the Mystery of Lyme and Chronic Disease: Pain, Fatigue, Memory and Concentration Problems, and Much More*. New York, NY: St. Martin's Press, 2013. Print.

Horton, Edward S., and Ronald L. Terjung. *Exercise, Nutrition, and Energy Metabolism*. New York: Macmillan, 1988. Print.

Jaminet, Paul, and Shou-Ching Jaminet. *Perfect Health Diet: Regain Health and Lose Weight by Eating the Way You Were Meant to Eat*. New York: Scribner, 2012. Print.

Kharrazian, Datis Randy. *Why Do I Still Have Thyroid Symptoms?* Garden City, NY: Morgan James Pub., 2009. Print.

LaValle, James B., and Stacy Lundin Yale. *Cracking the Metabolic Code: 9 Keys to Optimal Health*. North Bergen, NJ: Basic Health Publications, 2004. Print.

Lott, Joey. *Healing Chronic Lyme Disease Naturally*. 2nd ed., Archangel Ink, 2014. Print.

Lott, Joey. *The Mother of All Antioxidants: How Health Gurus Are Misleading You and What You Should Know about Glutathione*. Archangel Ink, 2014. Print.

Moalem, Sharon, and Matthew D. LaPlante. *Inheritance: How Our Genes Change Our Lives, and Our Lives Change Our Genes*. New York, NY: Grand Central Pub., 2014. Print.

Palmer, Michael. *Biochemical Pharmacology*. Hoboken, NJ: J. Wiley, 2012. Print.

Passer, Michael W., Ronald E. Smith, Michael L. Atkinson, John B. Mitchell, and Darwin W. Muir.

Psychology: Frontiers and Applications. Toronto: McGraw-Hill Ryerson, 2011. Print.

Pitchford, Paul. *Healing with Whole Foods: Asian Traditions and Modern Nutrition*. Berkeley, CA: North Atlantic, 2002. Print.

Schulman, Rifka C., MD, and Jeffrey I. Mechanick, MD. "Metabolic and Nutrition Support in the Chronic Critical Illness Syndrome." *American Association for Respiratory Care* (2012): Web.

Scott, B., S. St. Jeor, and M. Molini. "Evaluation of Criteria Used for Developing Predictive Equations for Resting Energy Expenditure." *Journal of the American Dietetic Association* 109.9 (2009): Web.

Stone, Matt. *Diet Recovery: Restoring Hormonal Health, Metabolism, Mood, and Your Relationship with Food.* Archangel Ink, 2013. Print.

Wahls, Terry L. *Minding My Mitochondria: How I Overcame Secondary Progressive Multiple Sclerosis (MS) and Got out of My Wheelchair*. IA City, IA: TZ Press, 2010. Print.

Websites

180 Degree Health, http://180degreehealth.com/blog/

Animal Pharm, http://drbganimalpharm.blogspot.ca/

Breaking the Vicious Cycle and the Specific Carb Diet, http://www.breakingtheviciouscycle.info/

Chris Kresser, http://chriskresser.com/

Critical Mas, http://criticalmas.com/

Dr. Lam: Body, Mind, Nutrition, https://www.drlam.com/

Dr. McDougall's Health and Medical Center, https://www.drmcdougall.com/

Dr. Wilson, http://drlwilson.com/

The FODMAP Friendly Food Program, http://fodmap.com/

The GAPS Diet, http://www.gapsdiet.com/

Healingwell.com: Community, Support, Resources, http://www.healingwell.com/

Klinghardt Academy, http://www.klinghardtacademy.com/

Mercola, http://www.mercola.com/

Ray Peat, http://raypeat.com/

CONNECT WITH ME

Here are a few ways you can connect with me:

Get my future books for FREE by signing up for my mailing list at itsnotjustlyme.com. No catches here.

Email me at yessington@itsnotjustlyme.com with your questions and feedback.

Kindly write a review on Amazon.com to help spread the word about this book.

Book a consultation with me. These are done over the phone or skype. Up to 60 minutes, all sessions are currently by donation.

All the best to you in your health endeavors.

Made in the USA
Middletown, DE
23 February 2017